The
Sleep Solution

A Comprehensive Guide to Overcoming Insomnia

By

Kimberly R. Pittman 2023

Table of Contents

INTRODUCTION

Do you constantly find yourself unable to fall asleep at night, staying awake and gazing at the ceiling? Do you have daytime fatigue and irritability, making it difficult for you to focus or perform at your best? If so, you might be one of the millions of people who experience insomnia globally.

People of all ages and socioeconomic backgrounds are susceptible to insomnia, a common sleep problem. Numerous things, such as stress, worry, depression, drugs, and lifestyle choices, might contribute to it. Whatever the underlying cause, the outcome is the same: a tiring cycle of insomnia that can leave you feeling rundown and ill.

But don't give up! You can beat insomnia and get the sound sleep your body and mind need using a number of techniques and treatments. There are choices to meet every person's needs and tastes, from straightforward lifestyle adjustments to natural cures to pharmaceuticals.

Therefore, read on if you're ready to recover the revitalizing power of a good night's sleep and are sick of tossing and turning all night. In this article, we'll look at the reasons for insomnia, how it may affect your health and happiness, and—most importantly—successful methods for dealing with this aggravating disease.

CHAPTER 1

Insomnia: What Is It?

One typical sleep issue is insomnia. You can experience difficulty going to sleep, staying asleep, or receiving good-quality sleep if you have insomnia. Even if you have the time and the ideal atmosphere for sound sleep, this still occurs. Your everyday tasks may be hindered by insomnia, which can also cause daytime sleepiness.

This may result in problems like:

• Daytime drowsiness and sluggishness

• A broad sense of being physically and mentally ill

• Alterations in mood, irritability, and anxiety

Additionally, the aforementioned problems may be causes, effects, or both of insomnia.

Stress, alterations in your routine, or your environment can all contribute to short-term sleeplessness. A few weeks or weeks may pass before it ends. Insomnia that is chronic (long-term) occurs three or more nights per week, lasts more than three months, and cannot be adequately accounted for by another medical condition.

Your doctor may inquire about your sleeping patterns and request that you keep a sleep diary in order to identify insomnia. Additionally, your healthcare professional may advise you to adopt healthy lifestyle practices like a regular sleep routine, cognitive behavioral therapy for insomnia, and the use of sleeping pills.

Your memory and attention span can be impacted by insomnia. Your risk of high blood pressure, coronary heart disease, diabetes, and cancer increases if you experience chronic sleeplessness.

Additionally, chronic illnesses like the following may be influenced by insomnia:

• Obesity

• Depression

Additionally, it can impair a person's effectiveness at work and school and restrict their capacity to carry out daily tasks.

What is Sleep?

Sleep is an organic condition of relaxation during which both the body and the mind experience a period of renewal and restoration. For physical and emotional health and well-being, it is a crucial physiological function. In order to preserve excellent health and well-being, sleep is a crucial physiological process. In addition to healing and renewing tissues, the body also consolidates memories and learning when sleeping and manages hormones and neurotransmitters.

The Cycle of Sleep

Multiple stages of sleep occur during the sleep cycle, each with its own distinct qualities and purposes. Comprehending the different factors that affect the type and duration of our sleep is crucial for comprehending the sleep cycle.

The two primary subtypes of sleep that comprise the sleep cycle are rapid eye movement (REM) sleep and non-rapid eye movement sleep.

Three levels further split NREM sleep:

Stage 1: This is when a person goes from being awake to asleep. It is a light state of sleep during which hypnic jerks or unexpected muscle spasms may occur.

Stage 2: During this stage of sleep, we are more deeply asleep and less conscious of our surroundings. The body temperature declines, the heart rate slows, and the breathing becomes more regular during this phase.

Stage 3: Also referred to as slow-wave sleep (SWS), this is the deepest stage of NREM sleep. The body heals and regenerates tissues during this stage of sleep while the brain consolidates learning and memory. It is the most restorative stage of sleep.

On the other side, REM sleep is distinguished by quick eye movements and elevated brain activity. We go through a time when we have vivid dreams. Memory consolidation and emotional regulation both depend on REM sleep.

The normal length of the sleep cycle is 90 minutes, and it occurs numerous times throughout the night.

Age, genetics, sleep disorders, medicine, and lifestyle elements, including stress, nutrition, and exercise, can all have an effect on the sleep cycle. Understanding the sleep cycle and making good sleep habits a priority will help us get more and better quality sleep, which will benefit our general health and well-being.

Why is Sleep so Crucial?

Our physical and mental health depends heavily on sleep, which is a biological necessity. It is a crucial component of daily life, just as crucial as maintaining a good diet and engaging in regular exercise. But why is rest so crucial? Let's look at some of the main causes.

Sleep is, first and foremost, important for physical well-being. The body boosts its immune system, regenerates tissues, and regulates hormone levels as you sleep. Obesity, heart disease, diabetes, and stroke have all been connected to sleep deprivation in studies.

Another important factor for mental wellness is sleep. The maintenance of healthy brain activity, including memory enlargement, problem-solving, and emotional control, depends on sleep. Chronic sleep loss has been associated with mental health illnesses like anxiety, depression, and other conditions.

Thirdly, getting enough sleep is crucial for productivity and performance. Getting adequate sleep might help you focus, concentrate, and make better decisions. Additionally, it increases energy levels and lessens weariness, which can enhance productivity and work effectiveness.

Last but not least, sleep is necessary for a high quality of life. We can feel revived, ready to take on the day, and refreshed after a restful night's sleep. Additionally, it improves our capacity for leisure pursuits and quality time with loved ones.

Getting enough sleep is important for maintaining good physical and mental health as well as performance and productivity. It's critical to emphasize sleep as a crucial component of a healthy lifestyle and to get assistance if you're having trouble falling or staying asleep.

Insomnia Types

By length, insomnia can be categorized as:

• **Transient, acute insomnia** is a short-term issue.

• **Long-term insomnia** can linger for several months or even years.

The causes are also classified by doctors:

Primary insomnia is a problem in and of itself.

Secondary insomnia is a repercussion of another medical condition.

They also categorize it according to severity:

• **Mild insomnia** is distinguished by a lack of sleep that causes fatigue.

• **Moderate insomnia** may impair day-to-day activities.

• Daily living is significantly impacted by severe sleeplessness.

When determining the kind of insomnia, doctors also take into account additional variables, such as whether the patient regularly wakes up too early or experiences difficulty:

• Nodding off

• Remaining in bed

• Receiving quality sleep

Hormones And Neurotransmitters' Function In Sleep

Neurotransmitters and hormones are crucial in controlling wakefulness and sleep. The timing and caliber of our sleep are regulated by these chemical messengers, which send signals to different regions of the brain and body.

Melatonin is one of the most crucial hormones in the control of sleep. The pineal gland releases this hormone in reaction to darkness, and its levels increase in the evening, alerting the body that it is time to go to bed.

Additionally, melatonin supports a normal sleep schedule by regulating the sleep-wake cycle.

Cortisol, another crucial hormone that plays a role in sleep regulation, is created by the adrenal gland in reaction to stress. Cortisol levels rise naturally in the morning to aid in promoting alertness and wakefulness and fall naturally in the evening to facilitate the start of sleep.

Neurotransmitters like serotonin, dopamine, and norepinephrine are also essential for controlling sleep. Dopamine is linked to motivation and reward, while serotonin is enmeshed in the control of mood, hunger, and sleep. Norepinephrine participates in the body's stress response and aids in promoting wakefulness and alertness.

Gamma-aminobutyric acid (GABA), a different neurotransmitter, is essential for controlling sleep. As an inhibitory neurotransmitter, it reduces brain activity and encourages relaxation and slumber.

Disorders of sleep can result from changes in neurotransmitter and hormone levels. For instance, low melatonin or GABA levels might make it arduous to fall asleep or stay asleep, but cortisol imbalances can mess with your sleep-wake cycle and make you inattentive.

We can better understand how hormones and neurotransmitters affect sleep regulation to find potential causes of sleep problems and create treatments that work. In addition to affecting hormone and neurotransmitter levels, lifestyle factors, including nutrition, exercise, and stress management, all have an impact on sleep quality and general well-being.

Symptoms of Insomnia

There are a variety of symptoms that you could feel if you have insomnia.

• It could take a little while for you to fall asleep after lying awake. Younger adults are more likely to experience this.

• Sleep might only be possible for brief periods of time. You can have many nighttime awakenings or spend most of the night awake. The majority of older persons are most commonly affected by this symptom.

• It's also typical to wake up too early in the morning and have trouble falling back to sleep.

• If you get poor-quality sleep, you could feel tired all day and wake up feeling unrested. You can also struggle to concentrate on routine duties. You may experience anxiety, depression, or irritability as a result of insomnia.

Keep a sleep journal or a list of any insomnia symptoms you may be experiencing. These notes should be given to a medical expert.

CHAPTER 2

The Effects of Sleeplessness on One's Health and Happiness

According to experts, sleep deprivation is a major contributing factor in car accidents.

Chronic sleeplessness or insomnia can have a serious negative effect on a person's health and well-being. Here are some ways that insomnia can have an impact on us:

Physical health: Obesity, diabetes, cardiovascular disease, and a weaker immune system are just a few of the physical health issues that insomnia has been related to. This is due to the critical function sleep plays in the body's capacity to regenerate and repair tissues, maintain hormone balance, and fortify the immune system.

Mental well-being: Chronic sleep deprivation has been associated with a higher risk of mental illness, including depression and anxiety. A vicious cycle of inadequate sleep and deteriorating mental health can result from insomnia, which can intensify the symptoms of pre-existing mental health issues.

Cognitive function: Sleep deprivation can affect one's capacity for memory, focus, and decision-making. Performance in school or the workplace, as well as the general quality of life, may be affected by this.

Emotional control: Insomnia can make it harder to control emotions, which can cause mood swings, irritation, and a decreased capacity to handle stress.

Social functioning: Lack of sleep can cause social retreat and decreased social interaction, which can affect interpersonal relationships and general social functioning.

Safety: Since people who are sleep deprived are more likely to have attention and reaction time failures, insomnia raises the risk of accidents and injuries.

In addition to interrupted sleep, insomnia can result in various problems, including:

• Daytime drowsiness or fatigue

• Anger, depression, or irritation

• Abdominal discomfort

• Lack of drive or energy

• Lack of attention and focus

• A lack of coordination, which can result in mistakes or accidents

• Concerns or anxiety related to sleeping

• Using sleeping pills or booze

• Headaches of tension

• Issues with working, studying, or socializing

Can I Avoid Having Insomnia?

Your doctor might advise you on measures you can take to improve your sleep and ward against persistent insomnia.

• To help you keep a regular sleep-wake cycle, develop healthy sleeping habits, and have a regular daytime schedule.

• Avoid consuming caffeine, nicotine, and alcohol within three hours of going to bed because they can interfere with your ability to do so.

CHAPTER 3

Risk Factors and The Causes

There are many different medical and psychological causes of insomnia. Frequently, a transient issue, such as transient stress, is the root reason.

In certain other cases, an underlying medical problem is the cause of the sleeplessness.

Typical causes include:

I. A Bedroom with Screen Technology: According to research, young individuals who use screens before night may have trouble sleeping.

Adults' sleep patterns may also be harmed by these devices. For instance, recreational usage after bedtime seems to raise the risk of sleeplessness.

Schedule or environmental changes can contribute to or increase your risk of sleeplessness. You can alter some risk factors, such as your employment or lifestyle. But you cannot change your age or your ancestry.

II. Age: Although insomnia can strike at any age, the likelihood that it will do so rises with age.

III. Genealogy and Genetics: Given that insomnia can run in families, your genes may increase your risk of developing the condition. Whether you are a deep sleeper or a light sleeper may also depend on your genes.

IV. The Environment or The Occupation: Your body follows a routine to determine when to go to sleep and when to be awake, which might be upset by the following:

• Night or shift work

• Nighttime commotion or light

• Uncomfortable temperatures, either high or low

V. Lifestyle: Your likelihood of having sleep issues may increase due to your way of life.

• Regularly altering your regular pattern, such as your sleep schedule

• Having sleep disturbances, such as frequently getting up to take care of an infant

• Sleeping a lot during the day.

• Engaging in insufficient physical activity throughout the day

• Utilizing caffeine, nicotine, alcohol, or illicit substances

• Using electronics or watching TV right before night

VI. Stress: Your risk of sleeplessness increases when you're under stress or worry about things like work or school, relationships, money, or the loss of a loved one.

Additionally, worrying about not getting enough sleep and keeping an eye on the time can increase your risk of developing insomnia or exacerbate it.

VII. Sex: Women are more odds-on than men to experience insomnia. Sleep issues may result from hormonal changes that happen during pregnancy and menopause.

VIII. Menopausal Effects: Sleeping problems are frequently caused by signs of various health problems or by changes in the natural world. For instance, hormonal changes during menopause might cause night sweats, which can keep you awake.

IX. Alzheimer's Disease: Sleep patterns are disturbed or altered in patients with Alzheimer's disease due to abnormalities in the brain.

X. Experiencing jet lag or any other alterations to the body's circadian clock.

XI. The bed is uncomfortable, and the room is too hot, cold, or noisy

XII. Providing care for a family member if it interferes with sleep

XIII. Experiencing nightmares or night terrors

XIV. Utilizing ecstasy or cocaine for recreational purposes.

XV. Some people experience insomnia as a result of stress

A person might be going through the following:

• Depression

• Anxiety

• Bipolar illness

• Schizophrenia

Other medical disorders that may interfere with sleep include:

• Tired legs syndrome

• An enlarged thyroid

• A sleep disorder

• GERD, or gastroesophageal reflux disease

• COPD, sometimes referred to as chronic obstructive pulmonary disease

• Persistent ache

Additionally, some people experience fatal familial insomnia, a rare genetic disease that makes it difficult to fall asleep and may possibly be fatal.

Diagnosis

Consult your doctor if not getting enough sleep is hurting your everyday activities. If you have problems falling asleep or staying asleep for at least three evenings a week, you might have insomnia. When it happens three or more evenings a week and lasts for three months or longer, insomnia is deemed chronic (long-term). To determine if your sleeplessness is contributing to any other health issues, your doctor may order additional testing.

Before visiting your doctor, it could be good to keep a sleep journal for one to two weeks. Your doctor can learn more about the issues you're experiencing and whether particular activities are interfering with your sleep by reviewing a sleep diary. Record your daily sleep, wake-up, and nap times in writing. Additionally, note when you consume caffeine or alcohol, when you exercise, and how drowsy you feel during the day.

Diagnostic Procedures

• A sleep study searches for further sleep issues such as narcolepsy, sleep apnea, and circadian rhythm disorders.

• Actigraphy examines your times of activity and rest and assesses how well you sleep. You must put on a little motion sensor for 3 to 14 days as part of this.

• Blood tests look for thyroid issues or other illnesses that could impair sleep.

Physical Examination and Medical History

Your doctor will be interested in knowing about your symptoms, risk factors, medical history, and family medical history. You might be questioned about your sleeping patterns in order to better understand your sleep issues, such as:

• How frequently and how long have you experienced sleep issues?

• When you sleep and wake up on workdays and on weekends.

• The amount of time it takes for you to fall asleep, how repeatedly you wake up at night, and how long it takes for you to fall asleep again.

• How rested and sleep-deprived you feel when you wake up and throughout the day.

• Whether you watch TV or use electronic gadgets before bed, the light from these sources may interfere with your sleep.

• Whether you snore loudly and frequently, wake up gasping, or experience breathlessness

Your healthcare professional could also inquire about the following to determine the root of your sleep issues:

• Experience any recent or ongoing health issues

• Consume any medications.

• Are you menstruating or expecting

• Use illegal drugs, alcohol, coffee, or nicotine

Your doctor will do a physical check-up to rule out any additional medical conditions that might be affecting your ability to sleep. They will examine your heart and lungs, listen to your heartbeat, and check for signs of sleep apnea, such as enlarged tonsils or a high neck circumference.

Treatment
1. Good Sleeping Practices

Try to adopt the following nighttime routines in addition to living a heart-healthy lifestyle. You may find it simpler to get to sleep and stay asleep if you practice these practices.

• **Create a sleeping-friendly bedroom.** Sleep in a peaceful, cool, and dark location. Avoid staring at electronics or watching TV since the light from these sources can interfere with your sleep-wake cycle.

• **Even on weekends, go to sleep and get up at around the same time each day.** Avoid schedule changes or other activities that can interfere with your sleep schedule if at all possible.

• **Refrain from consuming coffee, nicotine, or alcohol right before bed.** Alcohol can help you fall asleep more quickly, but your sleep may be lighter than usual as a result. You are more prone to experience nighttime awakenings as a result of this.

• **Exercise regularly during the day, at least 5 to 6 hours before retiring for the night.** Late-night exercise can make it more difficult to fall asleep.

• **Refrain from taking naps, especially in the afternoon.** You might sleep better at night if you do this.

• Follow a regular mealtime pattern and stay away from late-night feasts.

• **Drink in moderation before going to bed.** You might be able to sleep longer thanks to this and avoid using the restroom.

• **Acquire new stress-reduction techniques.** Establish a bedtime ritual that aids in your relaxation and winding down. Consider taking a hot bath, reading a book, or listening to relaxing music. In order to help you unwind, your doctor might also advise massage therapy, yoga, or meditation. Insomnia may also be improved by acupuncture, particularly in older persons.

• **Steer clear of over-the-counter and prescription medications** (such as some cold and allergy medications) that might interfere with sleep. Your healthcare practitioner can advise you on which medications won't interfere with your sleep.

2. Home Care Techniques

Many treatments and advice can support managing insomnia. They entail adjustments to:

Sleeping patterns

It can be advantageous to:

• Before going to bed, avoid using any screen-equipped devices.

• Start unwinding an hour before going to bed, for instance, by having a bath.

• Keep phones and other electronics away from the bedroom.

• Before going to bed, make sure the room is at a comfortable temperature.

• To make a space darker, use drapes or blackout shades.

Dietary Practices

• Avoid eating before bed. If you need to, have a healthy snack before going to bed.

• Prevent having a large meal within two to three hours of going to bed, though.

• Avoid drinking alcohol and caffeine after midnight.

• Eat a balanced diet to improve your overall health.

Optimum Health and Relaxation

• Practice deep breathing and relaxation techniques, especially before bed.

• Find a calming activity to do before bed, such as reading or listening to music.

• Even if you feel sleepy during the day, try to avoid taking a nap.

• If you experience any mental health problems, such as anxiety, seek medical attention.

CBT-I (Cognitive Behavioral Treatment) for Insomnia

A 6- to 8-week therapy program called CBT-I can teach you how to fall asleep more quickly and remain asleep longer.

This is frequently advised as the initial course of treatment for chronic insomnia and has the potential to be very successful.

A doctor, nurse, or therapist can provide CBT-I; it can be done in person, over the phone, or online. It consists of the following elements:

• You can feel less anxious about not being able to sleep, thanks to cognitive therapy.

• Meditation or relaxation treatment teaches you how to unwind and go off to sleep more quickly.

• Sleep education teaches you healthy sleeping practices.

• Sleep restriction therapy allows you to stay in bed for a set period of time, even if you can't fall asleep. This improves your ability to sleep at night over time. When you start to sleep better, you can extend your sleep time.

• Stimulus control therapy aids in maintaining a consistent cycle of sleep and waking so that you can associate lying in bed with sleeping. This means only napping when you're exhausted, getting up from bed if you have trouble sleeping, and only utilizing your bed for sleeping and having sex.

Additional Health Issues

One or more additional pillows might be used to elevate the upper body for anyone suffering from acid reflux or a cough.

Consult a physician for advice on how to treat pain, a cough, and any other symptoms that are keeping you up at night.

Medicines
• Medications on prescription

While some prescription sleep aids are intended for short-term usage, others are designed for longer-term use. Discuss the advantages and drawbacks of using medications for insomnia with your doctor.

Your risk of developing insomnia may also be increased by several prescription medications used to treat other medical disorders.

• **Drugs including zolpidem, zaleplon, and eszopiclone are benzodiazepine receptor agonists.** Anxiety is one of the side effects. Severe allergic reactions and engaging in activities while unconscious, such as eating, driving, or walking, are examples of rare side effects.

• **Medicines like ramelteon are melatonin receptor agonists.** Fatigue and dizziness are side effects. Some people have severe allergic reactions when they are asleep, which is a rare side effect of activities like eating, driving, or walking.

• **Suvorexant and other orexin receptor antagonists** are not advised for narcolepsy patients. Rare side effects could include the inability to move or talk for several minutes when you fall asleep or wake up, as well as engaging in activities while asleep, including eating, driving, or walking.

• If alternative therapies and medications haven't been successful, **benzodiazepines** may be administered.

Consult your doctor about the potential adverse effects of these medications, which may include disorientation, dizziness, and muscle weakness.

Additionally, benzodiazepines and other medications may interact in a harmful way. It should only be used for a few weeks because it can become habit-forming.

Supplement And Over-The-Counter Medications

Any OTC medications you are taking should be disclosed to your healthcare physician.

• Sleep aids that contain **antihistamines** are sold over the counter. Although you could feel tired after using these drugs, see your doctor before using them to cure your insomnia. For certain people, antihistamines can be dangerous.

• **Melatonin supplements** are manufactured copies of the melatonin sleep hormone. To enhance their sleep, many people use melatonin tablets. Melatonin has been studied. However, it has not yet been revealed to be a successful treatment for insomnia. Daytime sleepiness, headaches, upset stomach, and increasing depression are possible melatonin side effects. It may also have an impact on how your body regulates blood pressure, resulting in high or low blood pressure.

• While dietary supplements might be good for your health, there are also potential downsides. Before utilizing dietary supplements, consult your doctor.

Unapproved Medications

Sometimes medical professionals will prescribe drugs that are often used to treat other medical disorders but have not received U.S. approval. to treat insomnia. **Antipsychotics, anticonvulsants, and antidepressants are a few of these medications.**

CHAPTER 4

Natural Treatments for Sleeplessness
1. Teas and Herbal Supplements

Since ancient times, herbal dietary supplements and teas have been utilized as effective sleep aids. Here are some of the most sought-after herbal teas and medicines for treating insomnia:

• **Valerian root:** The natural sedative valerian root has been used for ages to induce sleep and relaxation. It can be purchased as a supplement and also made into tea.

• **Chamomile:** Chamomile is a well-liked herb that is frequently drunk as tea due to its relaxing and sleep-inducing qualities. It is thought to increase melatonin production, which controls the sleep-wake cycle.

• **Lavender:** Lavender is well-known for being soothing and relaxing. To encourage sleep, it is frequently used as an essential oil, added to bath water, or brewed into tea.

• **Passion Flower:** Research has revealed that this herbal sedative enhances sleep quality and lowers anxiety. It can be prepared into tea or bought as a supplement.

• **Lemon Balm:** Lemon balm is a natural sedative that can help you unwind and get a better night's sleep. It is frequently drunk as tea.

• **Ashwagandha:** Ashwagandha is an adaptogenic plant that can aid in promoting relaxation and lowering stress levels. It is thought to increase GABA synthesis, a neurotransmitter that encourages sleep.

While herbal pills and teas can be useful for supporting sound sleep, it's crucial to remember that they could also combine with other prescriptions and cause negative effects. Before utilizing any herbal supplements or teas, it is imperative to speak with a healthcare professional, especially if you have a previous medical condition or are taking medication.

2. Relaxation Methods Like Yoga and Meditation

Meditation and yoga are two powerful relaxation methods that can help you get more restful sleep and lessen the symptoms of insomnia. Here are some ways that yoga and meditation might enhance sleep:

• **Meditation:** To reach a state of peace and relaxation, meditation includes focusing attention on a single idea, thing, or action. By meditating before bed, you can calm your mind, ease stress and anxiety, and encourage sound sleep.

• **Yoga:** To encourage relaxation and lower stress, yoga combines physical postures, breathing exercises, and meditation. Gentle yoga positions can assist in increasing relaxation and reducing stress before bed, which will make it easier to get to sleep and remain asleep.

The following relaxation exercises can be included in your routine to encourage sound sleep:

• **Deep Breathing:** To promote relaxation and lower tension, deep breathing is a relaxation method that involves taking slow, deep breaths. Sit or lay down in a comfortable position and take a few deep breaths through your nose to fill your lungs with air. After a little period of holding your breath, slowly let it out through your mouth.

• **Progressive Muscle Relaxation:** Steadily relaxing the muscles is a technique that involves contracting and releasing various muscle groups in order to encourage relaxation and lessen tension. Start by tensing your toes and feet, maintaining the rigidity for a few seconds, and then letting it go to learn gradual muscle relaxation. Once you have tensed and relaxed every muscle in your body, move on to your calves, thighs, and so on.

• **Guided Imagery:** Guided imagery is a technique for promoting relaxation and lowering stress that involves employing mental images. Close your eyes and envision a serene setting, such as a beach or a forest, to practice guided imagery. Imagine the scene's sights, sounds, and aromas, and allow yourself to completely lose yourself in it.

Other Therapies

Your doctor might advise using light treatment to establish and keep your sleep-wake cycle regular. In order to receive this treatment, schedule time each day to sit in front of a light box that emits a bright light that is comparable to sunlight.

Sleep and the Effects of Light and Darkness

Since these environmental cues are so important in regulating the body's natural sleep-wake cycle, their effects on sleep are profound.

Melatonin is a hormone that helps people fall asleep. When exposed to light, especially blue light from electronics, melatonin production might be suppressed. It may be harder to get to sleep and stay asleep as a result of this upsetting the body's natural sleep-wake cycle. Bright light exposure in the evening or at night can also affect the quality of sleep, resulting in less rejuvenating and restorative sleep.

Darkness, on the other hand, encourages the creation of melatonin, which tells the body that it is time to go to bed. A quiet, dark sleeping environment can encourage relaxation and restfulness, improving the quality and length of sleep.

People who work nights or have irregular sleep cycles should pay particular attention to how light and darkness affect sleep. Bright light exposure at night can interfere with the body's natural sleep-wake cycle, making it harder to get to sleep and stay asleep during the day. In these situations, it's crucial to make the bedroom dark and quiet during the daytime, utilizing blackout curtains and white noise to encourage sleep.

The natural cycle of sleep and wakefulness can potentially be disturbed by using electronics right before bed.

To lessen the effect of blue light on melatonin production, experts advise avoiding electronic gadgets for at least an hour before sleeping or wearing blue light-blocking eyewear.

As a result of the important effects that light and darkness have on sleep, it is crucial to emphasize a peaceful, dark sleeping environment in order to encourage the best possible sleep quantity and quality. Avoiding exposure to strong light, especially in the evening and at night, can assist in regulating the body's normal sleep-wake cycle, resulting in more rejuvenating and restorative sleep.

The Advantages of Sound Sleep

Numerous advantages for our physical and mental health come from sound sleep. The following are a few of the main advantages of sound sleep:

• **Better Cognitive Performance:** Better cognitive performance is a result of getting enough sleep that is both restful and uninterrupted. It encourages learning and improves memory consolidation.

• **Enhanced Physical Performance:** Since sleep promotes muscle healing, repair, and growth, it is crucial for athletes and those who engage in physical exercise. Additionally, it enhances hand-eye coordination and reaction time.

• **Enhanced Immune System:** The body creates cytokines during deep sleep, a type of protein that aids in the defense against stress, illness, and inflammation. A restful night's sleep can improve the body's immunological response and serve as a defense against disease.

• **Improved Mood:** Getting enough sleep can help us feel better emotionally, lessen stress, worry, and despair, and make it easier for us to control our emotions. It encourages optimism and aids in controlling unpleasant moods and emotions.

• **Lowered Risk of Chronic Illnesses:** Sleep is essential for maintaining the balance of several hormones and neurotransmitters that affect our health. The chance of developing chronic illnesses, including heart disease, diabetes, and obesity, can be lowered by getting enough restorative sleep.

• **Increased Creativity:** A good night's sleep encourages original thought and problem-solving. It enables the brain to digest data, develop connections, and produce fresh concepts.

CONCLUSION

A typical issue is insomnia. It may be caused by a variety of problems, some of which may be related to physical or mental health. Some of the time, they are environmental or have to do with lifestyle choices like shift work, drinking alcohol, or caffeine.

Lack of sleep can bring about a range of issues, from minor fatigue to chronic sickness.

Anyone who consistently has difficulties sleeping and believes that it is interfering with their daily activities should consult a doctor, who can help ascertain the cause and make treatment recommendations.